I0446203

Eosinophilic Esophagitis Therapy & Diet

Mastering EOE Management Through Proactive Lifestyle Choices.

Title:
Eosinophilic Esophagitis Therapy & Diet

Subtitle
Mastering EOE Management Through Proactive Lifestyle Choices.

Copyright © 2023 by (Enola Cormier)

All rights reserved. No part of this publication may be reproduced, distributed, or transmitted in any form or by any means, including photocopying, recording, or other electronic or mechanical methods, without the prior written permission of the publisher, except in the case of brief quotations embodied in critical reviews and certain other non-commercial uses permitted by copyright law. For permission requests, write to the publisher, addressed at the address below.

Printed in the United States of America.

ISBN: 9798872272434

TABLE OF CONTENT

INTRODUCTION

The presence of an increased number of eosinophils, which are a type of white blood cell, in the lining of the esophagus, is the defining characteristic of eosinophilic esophagitis (EOE), which is a chronic inflammatory illness of the esophagus described by the acronym EOE. A wide variety of symptoms, such as trouble swallowing, chest pain, heartburn, and food impaction, can be brought on by this illness. An aberrant immunological response to particular meals is thought to be the causal factor behind EOE, even though the actual source of the condition is not completely understood.

Understanding Eosinophilic Esophagitis (EOE)

- **The Basics of EOE**

Eosinophilic Although esophagitis is a disorder that is not very common, the number of people who suffer from it has been steadily growing over the past several decades. Infiltration of eosinophils into the tissue of the esophagus, which results in inflammation and injury, is the defining characteristic of eosinophilic esophagitis (EOE). Eosinophils are a type of white blood cell that plays a role in allergy reactions. The number of eosinophils in the esophagus is a significant predictor of how the immune system reacts to specific stimuli.

- **Common Symptoms and Diagnosis**

EOE patients frequently have symptoms that are similar to those of other gastrointestinal conditions, making diagnosis difficult. Chest pain, chronic heartburn, trouble swallowing, and a feeling that food is stuck in the throat are some of the symptoms. To diagnose eosinophilic infiltration of the esophagus, a combination of endoscopy, biopsy, and medical history is usually used.

- **Link to Allergies and Atopic Conditions**

Atopic disorders, like eczema and asthma, are intimately linked to allergic problems, and those with a history of these conditions are more susceptible to EOE. This link points to a possible immune system malfunction, in which the body reacts negatively to some meals, causing the esophagus to become inflamed.

- **Treatment Approaches**

Corticosteroids are frequently used in traditional EOE therapies to lower inflammation. Nonetheless, the importance of nutrition in treating this illness is becoming more well-acknowledged. Reducing eosinophilic infiltration and managing symptoms have both been demonstrated to be achievable by identifying and removing particular dietary triggers.

Importance of Diet in Managing EOE

- **Diet as a Therapeutic Approach**

Understanding how nutrition affects EOE represents a paradigm shift in how it is managed. In contrast to other gastrointestinal disorders, where pharmaceuticals are frequently the main emphasis, EOE necessitates a more thorough examination of dietary components. Specific foods are common EOE triggers; reducing inflammation and symptom relief can be achieved with a specific dietary strategy.

- **Identifying Trigger Foods**

Finding particular trigger foods that worsen symptoms is the first step in controlling EOE with diet. An elimination diet is frequently used in this approach, in which possible allergens are methodically cut out of the diet and their reintroduction is closely watched to determine which foods are causing the problems.

- **Role of Allergy Testing**

Testing for allergies, such as blood and skin prick tests, might help identify putative dietary triggers. These examinations evaluate the immune system's reaction to particular allergens, offering important data for developing a customized dietary regimen. It's important to remember, though, that not all trigger foods may be identified by these tests, and clinical symptoms are still a major diagnostic component.

- **Elimination Diets and Their Effectiveness**

With elimination diets, common allergens like dairy, wheat, soy, and eggs are cut out of the diet for a predetermined amount of time. As a result, the esophagus can mend and the symptoms go away. These foods are then phased back one by one to pinpoint the precise triggers. The important role that nutrition plays in this disorder is highlighted by the success of elimination diets in addressing EOE.

- **Nutritional Considerations**

Making sure you're getting enough nutrients is essential while controlling EOE with food. Meeting dietary needs might be difficult when some food types are eliminated. Working with healthcare providers—dietitians included—to develop a well-balanced diet that addresses nutritional deficits and promotes general health is crucial.

- **Ongoing Management and Dietary Modifications**

Since EOE is a dynamic illness, dietary interventions may not always be as successful as they initially seem. Successful long-term management involves regular monitoring, working with healthcare specialists, and being willing to modify the diet based on individual reactions.

GETTING STARTED

Eosinophilic esophagitis (EOE) management requires a multidisciplinary strategy that begins with a comprehensive understanding of the problem, a correct diagnosis, and coordination with healthcare specialists. This is the first step in the path. In this process, one of the most important steps is to establish attainable objectives for dietary adjustments. This will ensure that the management plan is both sustainable and effective.

Diagnosing Eosinophilic Esophagitis

In order to initiate an effective management plan, it is essential to have a solid understanding of the symptoms and diagnostic methods associated with EOE.

Recognizing Symptoms:

The symptoms of EOE can sometimes be mistaken for other gastrointestinal problems, making diagnosis difficult. The initial approach is to identify the symptoms, which include food impaction, chronic heartburn, difficulty swallowing, and chest pain. Maintaining an in-depth symptom journal can be very beneficial for both patients and medical providers.

Medical Evaluation:

It is essential to seek a medical assessment if EOE is suspected. Gastroenterologists specialize in the diagnosis and treatment of digestive system illnesses, such as EOE. The diagnostic approach usually includes a thorough medical history, a physical examination, and an initial evaluation of symptoms.

Endoscopy and Biopsy:

An upper endoscopy, which includes passing a flexible tube through the mouth and examining the esophagus with a camera, is frequently required for a conclusive diagnosis. Biopsies are obtained from the lining of the esophagus during the procedure to assess the degree of eosinophilic infiltration. Confirmation of EOE is mostly dependent on these biopsies.

Histological Analysis:

Following the biopsies, the tissue is examined under a microscope by a pathologist as part of the histological analysis process. If there are increased amounts of eosinophils, this validates the diagnosis of EOE. The extent of eosinophilic infiltration aids in determining the illness's severity.

Rule Out Other Conditions:

Peptic strictures and gastroesophageal reflux disease (GERD) must be ruled out due to their similar symptoms to other gastrointestinal ailments. A precise diagnosis guarantees that the treatment strategy is customized for each EOE.

Consulting with Healthcare Professionals

The development of an all-encompassing strategy for the management of EOE requires close collaboration with professionals working in the healthcare industry. In order to handle the many facets of the problem, this means that a group of specialists will collaborate with one another.

Gastroenterologist:

The main medical practitioner engaged in the diagnosis and continuing care of endometriosis (EOE) is a gastroenterologist. They can help people with the diagnostic process, go over possible treatments, and keep an eye on their progress because they are knowledgeable about gastrointestinal problems.

Allergist/Immunologist:

Seeing as how strongly EOE and allergies are related, speaking with an allergist or immunologist can be helpful. A focused dietary plan can be developed with the assistance of allergy testing, which can help pinpoint particular food triggers.

Dietitian/Nutritionist:

Developing an EOE-friendly food plan can be greatly aided by the expertise of a certified dietitian or nutritionist who specializes in gastrointestinal diseases. They collaborate with people to create a workable and long-lasting plan for dietary modifications, taking into account individual needs, possible inadequacies, and nutritional requirements.

Primary Care Physician:

Working in tandem with a primary care physician is crucial for managing general health. They can help with general well-being monitoring, other health concerns, and making sure the EOE management plan is in line with the overall objectives of healthcare.

Psychologist/Counselor:

Mental health and general well-being can be impacted by chronic illnesses like EOE.

Speaking with a psychologist or counselor can help with coping mechanisms, emotional support, and understanding the psychological aspects of managing a chronic illness.

Setting Realistic Goals for Dietary Changes

To successfully embark on a new nutritional adventure, one must adopt a method that is both realistic and sustainable. The establishment of attainable goals is critical for achieving long-term success in the management of EOE through nutrition.

Educational Goals:

Start by learning about EOE, its causes, and how nutrition affects symptom management. People can choose their diet more intelligently if they are aware of the science underlying the illness.

Consultation and Collaboration:

One of the main objectives is to have open contact with healthcare experts. Frequent meetings with nutritionists, allergists, and gastroenterologists offer chances to talk about the status, resolve issues, and tweak the treatment plan as needed.

Gradual Dietary Changes:

Set targets for modest dietary adjustments rather than making big changes all at once. This method enables the body to adjust, and people are more likely to follow the new eating schedule in the long run.

Identifying Trigger Foods:

Eliminating and identifying trigger foods is one of the main objectives. This could entail monitoring dietary consumption and symptoms with a thorough food journal. Establishing a tight collaboration with healthcare specialists, particularly dietitians guarantees a methodical approach to recognizing and addressing trigger foods.

Balancing Nutritional Needs:

Make sure that dietary modifications don't jeopardize the necessary amount of nourishment. Work with a dietitian to develop a food plan that is well-balanced and satisfies EOE's limits while also meeting nutritional requirements.

Monitoring and Adjusting:

Establish objectives for consistent symptom monitoring, following a diet, and general well-being. The management strategy can be modified as necessary thanks to this continuous assessment. To adjust dietary adjustments to each person's unique response, flexibility is essential.

Incorporating Lifestyle Changes:

Understand that controlling EOE involves more than just dietary changes. Establishing objectives for lifestyle modifications like stress reduction, consistent exercise, and enough sleep—improves general well-being and supports nutritional therapies.

UNDERSTANDING THE EOE DIET

The condition known as eosinophilic esophagitis (EOE) necessitates a cautious approach to nutrition since particular foods have the potential to cause inflammatory responses in the esophagus. In this section, we will discuss the essential elements that make up the EOE diet. These elements include an overview of the nutritional strategy, foods that should be avoided, foods that are generally safe, and the significance of reading food labels to identify potential triggers.

Overview of the Eosinophilic Esophagitis Diet

The EOE diet is a treatment strategy designed to reduce esophageal inflammation by identifying and avoiding particular trigger foods. In contrast to other diets that concentrate on improving overall health or managing weight, the EOE diet is extremely customized and takes into consideration the distinct triggers and sensitivities of each person.

- **Targeted Elimination:**

Eliminating foods that cause an immunological reaction in the esophagus is the cornerstone of the EOE diet. An elimination diet is usually used in this approach when common allergens and possible triggers are cut out of the diet for a certain amount of time.

- **Gradual Reintroduction:**

Following a phase of restriction, foods are progressively added back one at a time while closely monitoring any symptoms that may arise. This stage assists in identifying particular trigger meals that might be causing symptoms of EOE.

- **Personalized Meal Plans:**

There is no one-size-fits-all EOE diet. It necessitates a tailored strategy that takes into account each person's dietary requirements, preferences, and sensitivities. Creating a balanced and long-lasting food plan requires close collaboration with a registered dietitian or other healthcare provider with expertise in EOE.

- **Long-Term Management:**

Dietary approaches to effectively manage EOE are a continuous effort. Dietary modifications may be required as our understanding of trigger foods advances and our unique sensitivities to them alter over time. Consultations with medical professionals regularly guarantee that the diet plan continues to be beneficial and promotes general health.

Foods to Avoid

Managing Eosinophilic Esophagitis requires identifying and avoiding trigger foods. Some dietary groups are frequently linked to EOE, even though individual trigger meals can differ.

- **Common Allergens:**

A significant number of people who have EOE demonstrate reactions to common allergens, such as dairy products, wheat, soy, eggs, nuts, and seafood. The elimination of these allergens is typically done during the beginning stages of the EOE diet to evaluate the effect that they have on symptoms.

- **Acidic and Spicy Foods:**

Foods that are acidic or spicy can aggravate the symptoms of EOE by irritating the esophagus. To lessen discomfort and inflammation, meals strong in acidity, tomatoes, citrus fruits, and hot peppers are frequently limited.

- **Processed and High-Fat Foods:**

It is possible for processed foods and foods that are heavy in fat to contribute to inflammation and make symptoms of EOE worse. In the EOE diet, it is usual practice to limit the consumption of fried foods, processed snacks, and dairy products that are high in fat.

- **Artificial Additives and Preservatives:**

Artificial additives and preservatives present in processed foods may cause sensitivities in certain EOE individuals. These consist of synthetic tastes and colors as well as certain chemical preservatives. Keeping an eye out for these possible triggers becomes imperative while reading food labels.

- **Gluten-Containing Grains:**

Grains including wheat, barley, and rye contain gluten, which is a common cause of EOE. During the first stages of the EOE diet, gluten-containing grains are frequently avoided and their reintroduction is closely regulated.

- **Food Additives and Stabilizers:**

Carrageenan and guar gum are two examples of stabilizers and additives in food that may exacerbate the symptoms of encephalitis. These ingredients are frequently present in processed foods, such as processed meats and some dairy substitutes.

Foods that are Generally Safe

Certain meals are generally well tolerated by people who have eosinophilic esophagitis, even though the EOE diet requires the elimination of certain foods that pose a trigger for the condition. To develop a meal plan that is both nutritious and well-balanced, these items serve as the basis.

Lean Proteins:

Although the EOE diet calls for avoiding certain trigger foods, most people with eosinophilic esophagitis may tolerate other foods. These meals form the basis of a well-rounded and satisfying meal plan.

Non-Acidic Fruits:

Bananas, melons, and pears are examples of non-acidic fruits that are frequently a part of an EOE diet. These fruits can increase overall dietary intake and are less prone to irritate the esophagus.

Vegetables:

In the EOE diet, most vegetables are seen as safe, particularly when steamed or prepared. Carrots, squash, and green leafy vegetables are a few types of veggies that are usually well tolerated.

Whole Grains:

Whole grains that do not contain gluten, such as rice, quinoa, and oats, are frequently incorporated into the EOE diet. There is no evidence that these grains cause inflammation in the esophagus, although they contain vital nutrients and fiber.

Dairy Alternatives:

Alternatives to dairy products, such as almond milk, rice milk, or oat milk, are frequently investigated by people who have EOE and are sensitive to dairy products. For this reason, it is necessary to select alternatives that do not include any additional allergies or preservatives.

Healthy Fats:

The EOE diet allows for the inclusion of foods that contain good fats, such as avocados, olive oil, and nuts (for those who can tolerate them). The consumption of these fats can help to contribute to a well-balanced meal plan as they are a source of critical nutrients.

Reading Food Labels for Potential Triggers

To successfully navigate the EOE diet, it is necessary to have a great awareness of food labels to identify potential allergies and triggers. Being able to read labels becomes an essential ability when it comes to making educated decisions and avoiding foods that could potentially make EOE symptoms worse.

Identifying Allergens:

Common allergens are mandated to be listed on food labels, which makes it simpler for people who have EOE to recognize probable allergens that could cause their symptoms. Certain foods, such as milk, eggs, peanuts, tree nuts, soy, wheat, fish, and shellfish, are examples of common allergies. When choosing foods that are safe for consumption, it is essential to check for these allergies.

Avoiding Additives and Preservatives:

Preservatives and additives included in processed meals can pose health risks to those with eating disorders. Inflammation may be exacerbated by carrageenan, artificial coloring, and specific chemical preservatives. Avoiding these additives can be achieved by carefully reading ingredient labels and selecting minimally processed meals.

Understanding Food Terminology:

It's crucial to understand food lingo when reading labels. Phrases such as "natural flavorings" or "modified food starch," for instance, may conceal possible triggers. When in doubt, consulting medical experts for clarification or consulting trustworthy sources can aid in understanding complicated ingredient lists.

Checking for Hidden Allergens:

Due to cross-contamination during processing, certain items could include hidden allergies. If a product is processed at a facility that also handles common allergens, manufacturers are obligated to publish this information. People who have EOE should use caution when using these goods to avoid unintentional exposure.

Monitoring Serving Sizes:

To avoid overeating meals that could be a trigger, it is essential to have a solid understanding of the appropriate portion sizes. Excessive consumption of a food item may result in symptoms, even if the food item is generally thought to be harmless. One of the factors that helps to the overall success of the EOE diet is paying attention to the size of the portions.

CREATING YOUR EOE DIET PLAN

To effectively manage symptoms and improve overall well-being, it is essential to develop a food plan that is both effective and sustainable for those who suffer from eosinophilic esophagitis (EOE). In this section, we will discuss the components that are essential to the process of developing a tailored EOE diet plan. These components include the design of the plan, the balancing of nutritional needs, and practical recommendations for meal preparation and planning.

Designing a Personalized Meal Plan

The process of developing a specific meal plan for EOE requires an approach that is both thorough and methodical. All of the individual's trigger foods, nutritional requirements, and personal tastes are taken into consideration when developing a customized diet plan. Developing a personalized EOE meal plan involves the following essential steps:

Identifying Trigger Foods:

Finding and removing trigger foods is the cornerstone of an EOE diet plan. Collaborate closely with medical specialists, such as nutritionists and allergists, to identify particular foods that aggravate symptoms and inflammation. Maintain a thorough food journal to monitor your nutritional intake and any reactions that may arise.

Elimination Phase:

Start with an elimination phase in which the diet is adjusted to exclude identified trigger items. During this stage, the esophagus might mend and the symptoms go away. Frequently occurring trigger foods, like dairy, gluten, and some fruits, can be temporarily avoided. Later in the procedure, this phase acts as a baseline for the reintroduction of foods.

Gradual Reintroduction:

Reintroduce foods one at a time following the elimination phase while keeping an eye out for any negative reactions. This stage facilitates the identification of particular trigger foods and offers a more sophisticated insight into personal sensitivities. Throughout this time, stay in constant contact with medical specialists to receive advice and assistance.

Balancing Variety and Nutrition:

Despite limitations, strive for a varied and well-rounded diet. Include a range of well-tolerated fruits, vegetables, lean proteins, and entire grains. To make sure that nutritional needs are satisfied, a dietitian can offer advice on substitutes and alternatives.

Consideration of Individual Preferences:

Understand that dietary modifications should take culture and personal preferences into account. A diet plan that accommodates individual preferences is more likely to be long-term maintainable. Try out a variety of dishes and meal combos to find options that you enjoy and find satisfying.

Regular Monitoring and Adjustments:

A customized EOE diet plan is dynamic, adapting over time to each person's unique needs and shifting sensitivity levels. Keep a close eye on your general health, dietary compliance, and symptoms. Be prompt in getting in touch with medical experts and modifying the eating plan as needed.

Balancing Nutritional Needs

One of the most important aspects of controlling eosinophilic esophagitis while following dietary limitations is ensuring that appropriate nutrition is maintained. Ensuring that individuals with EOE acquire the needed nutrients for their general health can be accomplished by balancing their dietary needs. Consider the following guidelines when attempting to strike a balance between the EOE diet's nutritional requirements:

- Working together with a Dietitian: It is essential to collaborate with a qualified dietitian who is an expert in gastrointestinal illnesses, including EOE. A dietitian may evaluate each person's unique nutritional needs, rectify any inadequacies, and offer advice on how to adhere to dietary limitations without sacrificing nutritional quality.

- Focus on Entire Foods: The EOE diet should place a high priority on whole, minimally processed foods. Whole foods are a great source of vitamins, minerals, and other vital nutrients without the added chemicals and preservatives that can make symptoms worse. For a well-rounded nutritional diet, include a range of fruits, vegetables, lean proteins, and whole grains.

- Sources of Calcium and Vitamin D: Dairy is a common cause of EOE, which makes it difficult to get enough calcium and vitamin D. Investigate other sources of these nutrients, such as supplements, leafy green vegetables, and fortified plant-based milk, as advised by a healthcare provider.

- Protein-Rich Substitutes: Make sure you're getting enough protein, which is an essential macronutrient for healthy muscles and general well-being. The EOE diet can contain lean proteins from fish, chicken, and plant-based foods like quinoa, lentils, and tofu. If dietary consumption is inadequate, protein supplements should be taken into consideration.

- Fiber and Healthy Digestive System: Include foods high in fiber to promote digestive health. Even while the EOE diet may limit some high-fiber items, you can still receive your recommended daily allowance of fiber from things like cooked veggies, some fruits, and whole grains without gluten. If more fiber is required, supplements could be suggested.

- Hydration: Maintain adequate hydration as it can help with digestion and is vital for general health. The best option is water, though herbal teas could also work. Steer clear of acidic and caffeinated drinks to help avoid esophageal inflammation.

- Monitoring Micronutrient Levels: It's critical to routinely check the levels of micronutrients, such as iron, zinc, and B vitamins. These levels may be impacted by dietary limitations and possible malabsorption problems. If inadequacies are found, medical specialists can offer the right supplements.

Meal Prep and Planning Tips

When it comes to properly implementing and maintaining the EOE diet, effective meal preparation and planning are two of the most important factors. A well-planned preparation not only lessens the possibility of unintentionally coming into contact with trigger foods but also guarantees that meals that are both nutritional and risk-free are easily available. In the context of eosinophilic esophagitis, the following suggestions for meal preparation and planning should be taken into consideration:

Freezing & Batch Cooking: Batch cooking makes it possible to prepare bigger amounts of nutritious meals that can be divided into portions and frozen for later use. A variety of frozen dinners are convenient and cut down on the amount of cooking that must be done every day.

Build a Go-To Recipe List: Make a list of recipes that work well together and can serve as mainstays for an EOE diet. These dishes ought to be tasty, nourishing, and simple to make. Having a repertoire of go-to meals makes meal planning easier and diet consistency increases.

Meal Preparation on the Weekend: Set aside a particular day of the week, like the weekend, to prepare meals. Make use of this time to prepare meals for the next week, chop veggies, and cook proteins. Having prepared items on hand simplifies cooking during hectic workdays.

Invest in Safe Kitchen Equipment: Purchase distinct kitchenware for making EOE-safe meals to avoid cross-contamination. Cookware, utensils, and cutting boards fall under this category. Additional steps to lower the risk of unintentional exposure include labeling containers and setting aside particular places in the kitchen for EOE-friendly foods.

Prepare for Social Situations: For those with EOE, going to social events and eating out might be difficult. Inform hosts or restaurant workers in advance of any dietary requirements to prepare for such scenarios. At social gatherings, bringing safe meals to share guarantees that EOE-friendly options are accessible.

Use EOE-Friendly Substitutes: Look for and include EOE-friendly alternatives to foods that trigger allergic reactions. For instance, recipes can utilize plant-based milk, non-dairy cheese, and gluten-free substitutes. Trying out different replacements guarantees a variety of tasty dishes.

Keep Up With EOE-Friendly Brands: Keep up with food brands and products that are EOE-friendly. Some producers focus on products that are EOE-friendly or allergen-free. Learn to trustworthy brands so that choosing handy and safe food products is easier.

Inform Friends and Family: Inform your close friends and family about the significance of the EOE diet. An environment that is more welcoming and inclusive can be produced by their comprehension and assistance. Talk about safe substitutes, foods that provoke reactions, and the importance of following the diet plan.

NAVIGATING SOCIAL SITUATIONS

Being a person who lives with eosinophilic esophagitis (EOE) can present a unique set of obstacles in social settings, particularly when it comes to eating out, communicating dietary requirements to other people, and taking part in social activities. The purpose of this section is to provide complete information on how to navigate certain social circumstances while controlling EOE. Additionally, to enhance the whole dining experience, this section will provide suggestions for recipes and culinary tips.

Dining Out with EOE

To have a safe and comfortable dining experience when dining out, people with Eosinophilic Esophagitis need to take proactive precautions, communicate effectively with restaurant workers, and carefully assess their menu options.

1. Investigating Restaurants: Check the menu and, if available, the allergen information before selecting a restaurant. These days, a lot of eateries offer online menus with allergy listings. Select restaurants that have a track record of honoring dietary requirements and disclosing ingredients.

2. Making a Reservation: Make the effort to give the restaurant a call in advance to go over your dietary requirements. This allows you to find out about particular menu items, any allergies, and whether the restaurant would fulfill special requests. Some eateries could even be open to altering menu items to meet your specific needs.

3. Clearly Expressing Dietary Restrictions:

4. Inform the server of your dietary limitations as soon as you arrive at the restaurant. Give a brief explanation of your Eosinophilic Esophagitis and a list of foods or ingredients that should be avoided as triggers. When

emphasizing the significance of avoiding particular allergens, be kind yet forceful.

5. Selecting Easy Recipes: Go for straightforward, minimally processed foods that are less likely to include unidentified allergies. Simple rice or potatoes, steaming veggies, and grilled proteins are frequently safer options. Steer clear of complicated marinades, sauces, and meals that have a lot of ingredients to lower the chance of unintentional exposure.

6. Bringing Safe Snacks: If there aren't many options at the restaurant, think about bringing a little snack that you know is safe

to eat. If there aren't many appropriate menu options, this precaution guarantees that you won't go hungry.

7. Developing Connections with Neighborhood Restaurants: It may be beneficial to cultivate a relationship with neighborhood restaurants. You may find that chefs and staff are more accommodating when they are aware of your dietary needs. You may improve your dining experiences by routinely going to places that are considerate of and accommodating to your needs.

8. Stay Alert at Buffets: Because of the possibility of cross-contamination, buffets

can be difficult for those with EOE. Ask questions about the ingredients and cooking techniques used in each dish if you're at an event that is served buffet style. To reduce the chance of cross-contact, think about arriving early.

Explaining Your Dietary Needs to Others

When in social circumstances, it is essential to communicate your nutritional requirements effectively. At any event, whether you are going to a potluck or dining at a friend's house, it is important to communicate your preferences to make sure that everyone participating has a pleasant and secure time.

- Inform Friends and Family: Invest some time in educating your close friends and family about food limitations and eosinophilic esophagitis. Talk about common allergies, foods that provoke reactions, and the significance of avoiding particular substances.

- Give precise instructions: Provide explicit instructions on what foods are safe for you to eat and what you should avoid. Make a list of foods or allergies that trigger you, and invite friends and family to contact you with any queries they may have about certain ingredients or recipes.

- Volunteer to Help With Meals: If you're invited to a friend's house for a meal, offer to help out by bringing one or two dishes that fit your dietary needs. This relieves the host of any possible tension while also guaranteeing that you have safe options.

- Bring EOE-Friendly Snacks: Bring your shareable EOE-friendly snacks to social events. This not only guarantees that you have safe options, but it also introduces delectable, allergy-friendly substitutes to others.

- Communicate Proactively: Don't wait to ask someone about your dietary requirements; instead, make an effort to let them know. Talking about your demands in advance makes people more receptive to your requests and shows that you are dedicated to managing EOE.

- Show Your Appreciation for Accommodations: Show your appreciation for the efforts made by others to meet your dietary requirements. Acknowledging their achievements encourages a cooperative and upbeat environment, which improves everyone's enjoyment of subsequent interactions.

Managing EOE in Social Gatherings

People who suffer from eosinophilic esophagitis may experience difficulties when attending social gatherings, regardless of whether they are held at someone's home or a public event. In a variety of social contexts, the following are some ways to manage EOE:

- Speaking with Hosts: Make sure you get in touch with the host well in advance if you plan to attend a party at their house. Declare what you need to eat, offer to bring something safe, and make sure the host knows about any dietary limitations. It can assist in providing a list of foods that provoke anxiety.

- Handling Potluck Events: Attending a potluck may be exciting and difficult at the same time. If you're attending a potluck, make sure there are safe options available for you by coordinating with the host. Think about providing food that you and others will both appreciate.

- Bringing EOE-Friendly Dishes: Bring EOE-friendly dishes to share at social events when the occasion calls for it. This guarantees that you have safe selections and also introduces others to delectable, allergen-free options.

- Establishing a "Safe Zone": Set aside a specific area for yourself at larger events. This may entail selecting a seat or location away from possible stressors so that you may enjoy the event in a worry-free and comfortable environment.

- Making Use of Discreet Meal Cards: You might want to draft discreet meal cards that list your dietary constraints in brief. When dining out or visiting gatherings, you can share this card with the hosts or servers, which will make it easier for them to meet your needs.

- Being Ready for Inquiries: Be ready for inquiries concerning your dietary requirements from friends, relatives, or acquaintances. Being prepared with a succinct but insightful explanation promotes understanding and aids in educating others.

RECIPE IDEAS AND COOKING TIPS

There is a mix of thoughtful ingredient selection, creative recipe development, and cooking procedures that preserve nutrients that are required to create meals that are both delicious and suitable for EOE. In this part, you will find a thorough guide on recipes, cooking techniques, and ideas for quick meals that are suitable for people with Eosinophilic Esophagitis (EOE). These can help you improve your culinary experience while also efficiently managing your condition.

EOE-Friendly Recipes

To create dishes that are suitable for EOE, it is necessary to carefully pick the components and think of creative ways to approach flavor. Following is a selection of dishes that are suitable for people who suffer from eosinophilic esophagitis:

- **Quinoa Salad with Roasted Vegetables:**

Ingredients:

- Olive oil
- Fresh herbs (basil, parsley)
- Quinoa
- Assorted vegetables (bell peppers, zucchini, cherry tomatoes)
- Lemon juice
- Salt and pepper to taste

Instructions:

- Follow the directions on the package to cook the quinoa.
- Add salt, pepper, and olive oil to roasted vegetables.
- Combine roasted vegetables with cooked quinoa.
- Add a drizzle of lemon juice, fresh herbs, and olive oil.

- **Grilled Lemon Herb Chicken:**

Ingredients:

- Garlic (minced)
- Fresh herbs (rosemary, thyme)
- Chicken breasts
- Lemon juice
- Olive oil

- Salt and pepper to taste

Instructions:

- Lemon juice, olive oil, minced garlic, fresh herbs, salt, and pepper are all used to marinate chicken.
- Cook on the grill until done, for a moist and tasty finish.

- **Vegetarian Stir-Fry with Tofu:**

Ingredients:

- Firm tofu
- Garlic (minced)
- Sesame oil
- Brown rice or rice noodles
- Mixed vegetables (broccoli, bell peppers, carrots)

- Soy sauce (low-sodium)

- Ginger (minced)

Instructions:

- Tofu should be pressed, cubed, and stir-fried till golden brown.

- Ginger and garlic minced are sautéed in sesame oil.

- Stir-fry the mixed vegetables and tofu in the pan until the vegetables become soft.

- Add low-sodium soy sauce and toss.

- Serve with rice noodles or brown rice.

- **Gluten-Free Banana Oat Muffins:**

Ingredients:

72

- Gluten-free oats
- Baking powder
- Cinnamon
- Vanilla extract
- Ripe bananas
- Eggs

Instructions:

- Tofu should be pressed, cubed, and stir-fried till golden brown.
- Ginger and garlic minced are sautéed in sesame oil.
- Stir-fry the mixed vegetables and tofu in the pan until the vegetables become soft.
- Add low-sodium soy sauce and toss.
- Serve with rice noodles or brown rice.

- **Roasted Sweet Potato and Chickpea Bowl:**

Ingredients:

- Sweet potatoes (cubed)
- Cumin
- Garlic powder
- Tahini sauce
- Chickpeas (drained and rinsed)
- Olive oil
- Smoked paprika

Instructions:

- Olive oil, smoked paprika, cumin, and garlic powder should be combined with sweet potatoes and chickpeas and then tossed together.

- Sweet potatoes should be roasted until they are soft.
- Immediately before serving, drizzle with tahini sauce.

Cooking Techniques to Retain Nutrients

Preserving the nutritional content of ingredients is crucial, particularly in the treatment of eosinophilic esophagitis. The following cooking methods preserve nutrients while bringing out the flavors:

Steaming:

Steaming is a gentle cooking method that preserves the natural flavors and nutrients of vegetables. It's particularly effective for vegetables like broccoli, carrots, and cauliflower.

Sautéing:

Ingredients are swiftly cooked in a tiny amount of oil during the sautéing process, keeping flavor and nutrients intact. Use healthful oils, such as coconut or olive oil, and flavor them with herbs and spices.

Grilling:

Grilling lets the surplus fat fall off while adding a smokey taste. For proteins like chicken, fish, and veggies, this is a great way to prepare them. To improve flavor, marinate ingredients ahead of time.

Baking:

Baking is a very flexible method that works well with grains, vegetables, and proteins. By boiling food in its fluids, it preserves nutrients, and you may flavor meals without causing EOE by adding herbs and spices.

Blending and Pureeing:

Blending and pureeing foods can create meals that are smooth and easy to swallow for people who have trouble with particular textures. For sauces, smoothies, and soups, this method works perfectly.

Herb and Citrus Infusion:

Herbs and citrus infusions can enhance flavors without depending on typical trigger components. Try experimenting with citrus fruits like lemon and lime, as well as fresh herbs like cilantro, mint, and basil.

Quick and Easy Meal Ideas

Having quick and simple meal ideas that fit the dietary criteria for Eosinophilic Esophagitis can be a lifesaver on hectic days. Here are some recommendations:

Grilled Chicken Salad:

Serve grilled chicken breasts with a simple dressing of lemon and olive oil, accompanied with a bed of mixed greens and cherry tomatoes.

Stir-Fried Quinoa Bowl:

For a quick and healthy dinner, stir-fry precooked quinoa with your preferred veggies, tofu or shrimp, and a small amount of gluten-free soy sauce.

Avocado and Chickpea Wrap:

Spread the avocado-canned chickpea mixture over a gluten-free wrap after mashing it. To make a delicious wrap, add lettuce, tomatoes, and a dab of olive oil.

Smoothie Bowl:

Mix frozen fruits, spinach, and your preferred dairy-free milk to create a superfood smoothie bowl. Add sliced bananas and EOE-friendly granola on top.

Egg Fried Rice:

For a simple and delicious egg fried rice, scramble eggs and combine with cooked rice, peas, carrots, and a small amount of gluten-free soy sauce.

Baked Salmon with Herbs:

Dredge salmon fillets in a mixture of lemon juice, fresh herbs, and olive oil. Serve the cooked salmon with steamed veggies when it has finished baking.

DEALING WITH CHALLENGES

The management of eosinophilic esophagitis (EOE) requires you to navigate a particular set of problems, such as overcoming setbacks, dealing with cravings, and seeking support from family and friends. In this section, we will discuss effective techniques for coping with these problems, and we will provide you with insights that you can put into practice to improve your health journey.

Overcoming Setbacks

In the process of controlling eosinophilic esophagitis, it is unavoidable to encounter any obstacles that may arise. It can be disheartening to have setbacks, whether they are the result of an inadvertent exposure to trigger foods, an exacerbation of symptoms, or difficulties in following guidelines on diet. Nevertheless, it is of the utmost importance to view failures as chances for learning and to cultivate resilience in the face of many kinds of difficulties.

- **Understanding Triggers:**

Consider the situations that failed. Determine which particular foods or circumstances served as a trigger for the setback. Having this knowledge will enable you to minimize similar problems and make better decisions in the future.

- **Reassessing Your Approach:**

Take time to reconsider how you are handling EOE. To examine and make any necessary modifications to your food plan, think about collaborating with healthcare specialists like allergists or dietitians. Using a cooperative and well-informed approach will help your management strategy work better.

- **Learning from Experiences:**

Every obstacle offers a chance to improve and gain knowledge. Take advantage of setbacks to refine your management strategy and gain a deeper understanding of your body's reactions. Maintain a thorough journal of your experiences, highlighting any patterns or trends that might be causing obstacles.

- **Cultivating Resilience:**

To develop resilience, it is important to acknowledge that failures are an inevitable part of the path. You should concentrate on the positive parts of your management efforts as well as the success that you have accomplished. Through the cultivation of resilience, one can recover from failures with a revitalized feeling of determination and dedication to their health.

- **Utilizing Support Systems:**

In times of difficulty, it is important to seek assistance from your healthcare team, friends, or support groups. It is possible to gain significant insights and emotional support by talking about difficulties with other people who can understand and empathize with you. Just keep in mind that you are not traveling this path alone and that there are tools available to assist you in overcoming obstacles along the way.

Managing Cravings and Food Temptations

Individuals who are managing eosinophilic esophagitis may experience difficulties in the form of cravings and temptations related to food. To successfully resist the impulse to indulge in trigger foods, you will need to engage in strategic planning and make a commitment to putting your health first.

Finding the Causes of Cravings:

Spend some time figuring out what causes your cravings. Is there a particular flavor, texture, or sentimental connection? You can deal with cravings more skillfully if you know what causes them in the first place.

Investigating EOE-Friendly Substitutes: Instead of dwelling on the foods you are unable to consume, investigate EOE-friendly substitutes that fulfill your cravings. For instance, try desserts made with fruits, alternative flours, or naturally sweetened options if you're craving something sweet.

Adding Diversity to Your Meals: To reduce emotions of deprivation, add variety to your diet. Try out new dishes, flavors, and culinary traditions that fit your dietary constraints. A menu that is interesting and varied helps lessen the urge for off-limits things.

Preparing Ahead for Tempting Circumstances: Recognize potential triggering points and make appropriate plans in advance. Having a plan in place can help you get through stressful situations like going to social gatherings, eating out, or giving in to cravings without sacrificing your nutritional objectives.

Engaging in mindful eating can help you become more conscious of the foods you choose to eat and the habits you have. Savor the flavors, textures, and scents of your food as you become more aware of your senses. Eating mindfully can increase contentment and decrease the craving for bad foods.

Celebrate Non-Food Prizes: Instead of using food as a reward, concentrate on using non-food rewards to mark accomplishments and significant anniversaries. This could be indulging in a favorite pastime, spoiling oneself, or pursuing interests that make you happy and fulfilled.

Seeking Support from Family and Friends

To properly manage eosinophilic esophagitis, it is essential to have the support of other people, including family and friends. In addition to providing a sense of community and emotional support, the establishment of a solid support system can also assist in practical matters.

Teaching Your Support System: Spend some time teaching your loved ones about eosinophilic esophagitis and the dietary limitations that come with it. Give them links to articles, websites, or information from your medical team so they may learn about the difficulties you face.

Expressing Your Requirements Clearly:

Inform your support system of your demands and limitations clearly and concisely. Open communication promotes understanding and collaboration, whether it is when talking about trigger foods, preferred cooking techniques, or the significance of preventing cross-contamination.

Including Loved Ones in Meal Planning: Include your family members in the process of organizing meals. Work together to develop meals that are EOE-friendly, experiment with new ingredients, and come up with inventive substitutes. This not only helps you maintain stronger relationships with your support system, but it also turns mealtimes into a fun, social occasion.

Thanking Family and Friends for Support: Thank your family and friends for their support. Express gratitude for their attempts to meet your dietary requirements and acknowledge the benefits of their comprehension. A nurturing atmosphere makes a big difference in your general well-being.

Joining EOE Support Groups: If you suffer from Eosinophilic Esophagitis, you might want to check out in-person or online support groups. Making connections with people who have gone through similar things to you can give you a sense of community and insightful perspectives. These communities frequently provide forums for asking for guidance, sharing triumphs, and trading advice.

Presenting Prospects for Participation:

Give your network of supporters the chance to actively engage in managing your EOE. This may be asking them to go to medical visits with you, try new EOE-friendly recipes, or take part in awareness campaigns. Including family members promotes a sense of cooperation and shared accountability.

MONITORING YOUR PROGRESS

The effective management of eosinophilic esophagitis is a dynamic approach that includes monitoring your progress, gaining an understanding of how your body reacts, and making any required alterations to your dietary plan. In this section, we will discuss practical ways for charting your trip, such as keeping a food journal, monitoring symptoms and reactions, and making adjustments to your diet based on the information you gather.

Keeping a Food Diary

One useful tool for people treating eosinophilic esophagitis is a food diary. It acts as a thorough log of your food consumption, symptoms, and general health. Maintaining an in-depth food journal can assist you in recognizing trends, stressors, and opportunities for enhancement in your management strategy.

Tracking Daily Food Intake: To begin, make a note of everything you consume during the day. Make sure you write down all of the ingredients, serving quantities, and cooking techniques. Add drinks, snacks, and any supplements or prescription drugs you may be taking.

Meal Timing: Keep a journal of the times you eat and snack. Make a note of any changes or anomalies in your dietary routine. There are situations where timing affects symptoms, and seeing patterns can reveal possible triggers.

Recording Symptoms and Responses: Keep a record of your food consumption as well as any symptoms or reactions you encounter. This covers the beginning and length of the symptoms, their severity, and any elements that might have influenced your responses. Heartburn, chest pain, and difficulty swallowing are common signs of EOE.

Tracking Hydration: Record the amount of water you consumed during the day. Drinking enough water is vital for good health, and dehydration can occasionally make EOE symptoms worse. Keep track of the amount of water you drink and any changes to your hydration routine.

Beyond what you eat and drink, take into account environmental factors that might affect your symptoms. Take note of weather variations, allergy exposure, stress levels, and other outside influences. These specifics can help provide a more thorough insight into how you manage your EOE.

Considering Emotional Health: Include in your food journal thoughtful observations on your mental health. Take note of any instances of stress, anxiety, or other emotions you may be feeling. Stress and emotional variables can affect digestive health.

Using Technology to Make Things Convenient: Use technology to streamline the procedure. Numerous applications and web resources are available for monitoring dietary consumption and symptoms. These technologies frequently have reporting and trend visualization capabilities.

Tracking Symptoms and Reactions

Within the context of the care of eosinophilic esophagitis, the monitoring of symptoms and reactions is an essential component. Through the process of rigorously tracking your body's responses, you will be able to identify foods that trigger your symptoms, evaluate the efficacy of your dietary plan, and improve your ability to communicate with various members of your healthcare team.

Recording the Beginning and End of Symptoms: When symptoms arise, record the beginning and end of the symptoms. This data can help you determine when reactions are most likely to occur and can direct food plan modifications.

Measuring Symptom Intensity: Using a scale ranging from moderate to severe, indicate the degree of your symptoms. This subjective evaluation can help provide a more accurate picture of how particular foods or circumstances affect your health.

Finding Trigger Foods: Keep an eye out for trends connecting particular foods or ingredients to the start of symptoms. Finding your trigger foods is a crucial first step in fine-tuning your diet. Certain proteins present in dairy, wheat, eggs, and other foods are common EOE causes.

Observing Symptom Changes Over Time: Keep an eye on how your symptoms alter over time. Are symptoms getting milder or more frequent? By monitoring any patterns in your symptoms, you and your medical team can assess how well your current treatment strategy is working.

Interacting with Medical Professionals: During follow-up visits, discuss your symptoms and reaction log with your medical team. With this data, they can evaluate your progress, offer well-informed suggestions, and modify your management plan as necessary.

Recognizing External Influences: Take into account any outside variables that can affect your symptoms. EOE symptoms might be impacted by stress, allergens in the environment, and prescription changes. You can attempt to manage these factors more skillfully if you are aware of them.

Making Use of Visual Aids: Draw charts or graphs to illustrate your symptom patterns. Determining links between particular foods, environmental circumstances, and the development of symptoms might be facilitated by visualizing trends.

Adjusting Your Diet Based on Progress

The management of eosinophilic esophagitis is a dynamic and continuing process that involves making intelligent adjustments to your diet based on your progress while managing the condition. As you keep note of the foods you consume and the symptoms you experience, you will be able to work together with your healthcare team to make specific adjustments that will improve your overall health.

- Examining Food Diary Entries: To spot trends and connections, go over your food diary entries regularly. Examine any patterns in the onset, severity, and length of the symptoms, as well as any possible triggers.

Making wise modifications is based on the information provided here.

- Consulting with Medical Experts: Arrange routine meetings to go over your progress with your medical team. Provide your diet journal, symptom log, and any health-related observations. This cooperative strategy enables medical practitioners to offer customized advice and suggestions.

- Food Reintroduction Gradually: If you're thinking about reintroducing particular foods because your symptoms have eased, take your time. Start slowly and pay attention to how your body reacts. This methodical technique reduces the possibility of causing symptoms and aids in the identification of tolerance levels.

- Trying Different Cooking Techniques: Investigate various cooking techniques for foods that stimulate reactions. Certain foods can often be made more palatable by altering the way they are prepared. For instance, it could be simpler for the digestive system to simmer veggies rather than eat them raw.

- Trying Other Foods: See what happens when you try different ingredients that fit your dietary constraints. Common trigger foods have many available replacements. Try lactose-free or plant-based milk substitutes, for example, if dairy is a trigger.

- Thinking About Allergen Testing: Talk to your medical team about the potential for allergen testing. Testing for allergens can assist in determining which foods may be causing your problems. You can use this knowledge to fine-tune your diet and lower your chance of coming into contact with trigger items.

- Putting Changes into Practice: In addition to food changes, think about making lifestyle changes that could improve your general health. This could involve practicing stress reduction strategies, drinking enough water, and fitting regular exercise into your schedule.

- Tracking Long-Term Progress: Acknowledge that managing eosinophilic esophagitis is a long-term process. Keep a close eye on your development, acknowledge minor accomplishments, and don't hesitate to make changes when necessary. Maintaining long-term success typically requires a mix of lifestyle changes, diet compliance, and continuing support from medical specialists.

Lifestyle and Dietary Maintenance

The effective management of eosinophilic disorder In addition to food limitations, esophagitis requires adopting a holistic approach to lifestyle and dietary management to be effectively managed successfully. In this section, we will discuss the most important aspects of this strategy, such as the incorporation of physical activity, stress management, and long-term nutritional plans to support your general well-being.

Incorporating Physical Activity

Physical activity plays a vital role in maintaining overall health, and for individuals with Eosinophilic Esophagitis, it can contribute to improved digestion, reduced stress, and enhanced well-being. Here are some considerations for incorporating physical activity into your routine:

- Select Pleasurable Activities: Choose enjoyable physical pursuits. Finding activities that you enjoy doing, whether it's dancing, yoga, swimming, or walking, enhances the chances that you'll maintain a regular fitness schedule.

- Begin Gradually: If you've never worked out before or haven't been active in a while, begin slowly. As your fitness level rises, start with low-intensity, short-duration exercises and gradually increase them. This methodical approach reduces the possibility of inducing symptoms.

- Choose Low-Impact Exercises: Take into account low-impact workouts that are easy on the digestive tract. Walking, stationary bike, and swimming are a few well-tolerated activities that can be tailored to your fitness level.

- Investigate Attentive Movement Techniques: Take up tai chi or yoga as examples of mindful movement. These exercises stress relaxation, flexibility, and mental health in addition to improving physical fitness.

- Make Consistency a Priority: When it comes to physical activity, consistency is essential. Strive for consistent, moderate activity instead of sporadic, hard sessions. Long-term health benefits and sustainability are often higher with this technique.

- Pay Attention to Your Body: Observe how your body reacts to physical activity. Adjust your schedule if specific activities or intensities cause symptoms. Finding a balance between continuing your activity and avoiding things that could make your EOE symptoms worse is crucial.

- Speak with Healthcare Professionals: If you have any concerns or pre-existing medical conditions, speak with your healthcare team before beginning a new fitness program. Depending on your unique health situation, they can offer advice on appropriate activities and safety measures.

Stress Management for EOE

The symptoms of eosinophilic esophagitis can be made worse by stress, which is why stress management is a vital component of long-term health and wellness. It is possible to have a good impact on both your mental and physical health by incorporating stress-reduction activities into your daily routine:

- Develop a calm and concentrated mind by engaging in mindfulness and meditation practices. These methods can be very beneficial for lowering tension and encouraging calm. Think about including quick mindfulness activities in your everyday schedule.

- Practice Deep Breathing: To help you relax and reduce tension, practice deep breathing. Regular use of methods like guided breathing exercises or diaphragmatic breathing is recommended, particularly during times of increased stress.

- Discover the benefits of progressive muscle relaxation, a method that entails methodically tensing and relaxing various muscle groups. This technique aids in the physical release of tension and may assist in reducing stress in general.

- Frequent Physical Activity: Physical activity is important for stress management in addition to being good for one's physical health. Choose a hobby or pastime you enjoy, and incorporate it regularly into your schedule.

- Setting Boundaries: To control stressors in your daily life, establish unambiguous boundaries. Setting priorities for your work, learning when to say no, and knowing when to take a break are some examples of how to do this. Setting up appropriate boundaries is essential to preserving equilibrium.

- Seeking Emotional Support: To get emotional support, get in touch with loved ones, friends, or support organizations. Talking to people who are aware of the difficulties in controlling eosinophilic esophagitis about your experiences and emotions can be consoling and lessen feelings of loneliness.

- Professional Counseling or Therapy: To learn more about coping processes and stress management techniques, think about obtaining professional counseling or therapy. A mental health specialist can offer tailored direction and assistance in managing stressors.

- Including Relaxation Techniques: Investigate several methods of relaxation, such as aromatherapy, taking warm baths, or relaxing to relaxing music. You can include these techniques into your everyday routine to help you de-stress and have moments of relaxation.

Long-Term Dietary Strategies

Particularly important for people who suffer from eosinophilic esophagitis is the maintenance of a long-term approach to the control of their food. Take into consideration the following strategies as you continue on your path to maintain a diet that is both pleasing and healthy:

- Frequent Examine of Dietary Plan: Arrange for your healthcare team to review your dietary plan regularly. Periodic assessments enable required adjustments to be made, as your symptoms and triggers may change over time.

- Integration of Diverse Foods: Strive for a diet rich in a range of nutrients and well-rounded. Try experimenting with meals that fit your dietary requirements and make sure you are getting all the vitamins and minerals you need.

- Experimentation with New Recipes: Try out different recipes to keep your diet pleasurable and interesting. To broaden your culinary expertise, look for cookbooks or internet resources that are EOE-friendly and offer inventive yet secure recipes.

- Watching Trigger Meals: Be aware of any changes in your body's reaction to particular substances and continue to keep a close eye on trigger foods. Maintaining this awareness is essential to customizing your diet to meet your demands as they change.

- Foods Can Be Gradually Reintroduced: If your symptoms are under control, you might want to think about reintroducing some foods gradually. Implement a methodical approach in close collaboration with your healthcare team, starting with tiny doses and closely monitoring your body's reaction.

- Dietician Consultation: If you have any questions about Eosinophilic Esophagitis, think about scheduling a consultation with a certified dietitian. A dietitian may offer individualized advice, assist in identifying nutritional gaps, and provide helpful hints for keeping a diet that is both balanced and fulfilling.

- Social Support for Dietary Decisions: Let people know what you need to eat by telling your friends, family, and neighbors. Creating a welcoming atmosphere makes it possible for social events and shared meals to be stress-free and pleasurable.

- Continued Education and Awareness: Remain up to date on nutritional approaches and developments in the treatment of eosinophilic esophagitis. You can make wise decisions regarding your health and well-being by continuing your education.

- Celebrate Progress and Milestones: Take note of and commemorate the accomplishments along the way. Acknowledging successes, whether they involve growing your food choices or effectively handling a difficult situation, promotes a positive outlook and reaffirms your dedication to long-term well-being.

CONCLUSION

As we come to the end of this management guide for Eosinophilic Esophagitis (EOE), it's necessary to take stock of where we've come from, acknowledge our accomplishments, and look forward to what lies ahead. We'll talk about the importance of accepting a positive outlook for the future, cultivating a happy mindset, and recognizing your accomplishments in this part.

Honoring Achievements

Acknowledging accomplishments, regardless of their magnitude, is an essential component of handling Eosinophilic Esophagitis. Recognizing and applauding accomplishments helps to foster a positive and driven mindset. The path is full of obstacles, changes, and moments of perseverance. The following are important things to remember:

Recognizing Progress: Give due recognition to the advancements achieved in the treatment of eosinophilic esophagitis. Every accomplishment is a step closer to improved health, whether it be recognizing trigger foods, sticking to dietary restrictions, or changing one's lifestyle.

Acknowledging Adaptive Tactics: Appreciate the coping techniques and adaptive strategies you've acquired throughout the journey. These tactics, which range from developing EOE-friendly meals to confidently handling social situations, demonstrate perseverance and ingenuity in the face of difficulties.

Emphasizing Personal Development: Reflect on the development you have experienced personally during the trip. People who have to deal with a chronic illness such as eosinophilic esophagitis frequently need to develop tolerance, fortitude, and a better awareness of their bodies. Acknowledge and rejoice in this development.

Thank You for Your Support: Thank you for the help that family, friends, medical professionals, and support groups have provided. The management of Eosinophilic Esophagitis is greatly aided by the cooperative efforts of a supportive network.

Encouraging Thinking Alterations: Acknowledge and applaud beneficial shifts in viewpoint and mindset. Developing an empowerment attitude is often necessary to overcome obstacles, allowing people to feel more in charge of their health and equipped to handle the intricacies of eosinophilic esophagitis.

Accepting Self-Care Practices: Be proud of the self-care activities you include in your daily life. These self-care routines, which include setting aside time for rest, partaking in fun pursuits, and placing a high value on mental health, are essential to long-term well-being.

People with Eosinophilic Esophagitis can develop a sense of accomplishment, increase motivation, and create a positive attitude on their continuing journey by actively recognizing and celebrating their accomplishments.

To sum up, the process of addressing eosinophilic esophagitis is dynamic and always changing. Appreciating accomplishments, no matter how minor helps to maintain a positive outlook, and planning for the future entails remaining informed, actively engaging in one's health journey, and cultivating hope. As people persevere in managing the intricacies of

Eosinophilic Esophagitis, they might find solace in their accomplishments, the encouragement of their social circle, and the possibility of continuous enhancements in their general health and welfare.

www.ingramcontent.com/pod-product-compliance
Lightning Source LLC
Chambersburg PA
CBHW062314290526
45794CB00005B/1801